Distance
and
Disconnection

Author: Hannes van Zyl

The Hidden Struggles of Christian Men Away from Home

Distance and Disconnection: The Hidden Struggles of Christian Men Away from Home

Email: Authorhannesvanzyl@gmail.com

Pretoria

Gauteng

South Africa

Contents

Introduction

We all have insecurities that can sometimes feel overwhelming, but it's crucial to express them in a healthy and constructive way. If you're feeling uneasy about the long-distance nature of your relationship, it's important to avoid letting those feelings slip into passive-aggressive behaviour, which can be damaging. When you fail to discuss your emotions in a calm and open manner, it can lead to the creation of a toxic environment in your relationship. It's essential to voice your concerns to your partner and seek reassurance in a positive, supportive manner. Approach them for support with respect and understanding, and in turn, offer your trust when there's no valid reason for suspicion. Trust is a fundamental pillar in any relationship, and it becomes even more critical in long-distance dynamics where uncertainty can easily take root. Another significant challenge in long-distance relationships is managing differing expectations. A major indicator that your relationship may be facing difficulties is when you stop sharing common goals and dreams. It's perfectly normal for couples to have different perspectives on various matters; however, it becomes problematic when you lack shared objectives. This disconnect can lead to emotional distance, which ultimately weakens your bond. Infidelity is an especially serious deal breaker in long-distance relationships, where temptation may be heightened due to physical separation. It's vital to be honest with yourself about your emotions and the reality of your situation. When couples are apart, they may find themselves drifting and seeking happiness elsewhere. While it's absolutely acceptable to pursue individual interests and passions, be cautious not to neglect your partner in the process. Consider revisiting the activities you once enjoyed together to help keep the spark alive, even amid the challenges of distance. If you find yourself confiding in friends, "my long-distance relationship is draining me," it could be a signal that either you or your partner isn't investing the necessary effort to sustain the connection. It's entirely normal to experience such feelings occasionally, especially when physical distance limits your interactions. However, if you genuinely want to strengthen your bond, there are always strategies you can implement to enhance your relationship. Unhappiness can significantly impact a long-distance relationship. If you're feeling down or disconnected, take some time to reflect on the reasons behind these feelings. It's perfectly okay to seek support from your partner, but if they are contributing to your unhappiness, maintaining the relationship may become increasingly challenging. If certain issues are causing you distress, it's important to discuss them openly with your partner and collaborate on finding solutions together. Ignoring these problems can lead to serious consequences and further emotional rifts in a long-distance relationship. In such relationships, feelings can gradually fade if both partners don't actively work to sustain their connection and emotional investment. Couples may struggle when they can no longer relate to one another, a situation that can ultimately determine the future of the relationship. If you feel like you've grown apart over time, consider making an effort to reconnect, or have an honest conversation about whether it's best to go your separate ways. Regular, meaningful communication is absolutely crucial for maintaining the relationship, especially when faced with physical distance. It helps keep you linked and ensures that the relationship can endure. Without consistent communication, the relationship may weaken, as sporadic contact is a primary reason for the breakdown of long-distance relationships. The stability of the relationship may become compromised if partners start engaging with others outside of it, regardless of the distance separating them. A simple gesture, like sending a quick message or making a phone call, can provide much-needed reassurance and help prevent the relationship from unravelling. Be creative in reaching out and actively demonstrate to your partner the effort and attention they truly deserve. Taking the time to show your love and commitment can make a significant difference in nurturing your long-distance relationship.

Acknowledgements

To all of you who are navigating the often intricate and multifaceted complexities of relationships, marriages, or any form of commitment while one partner finds themselves working far away or overseas, I want to take a moment to sincerely commend your unwavering dedication and remarkable resilience. It is truly inspiring to witness the strength you all exhibit during these challenging times. I sincerely hope that your hearts, along with every other aspect of your relationship, remain not only strong but also united enough to endure this difficult and trying period.

Throughout my years of working with individuals in overseas jobs, I have observed a recurring pattern that many face: such situations rarely remain short-term. Instead, they often evolve into a long-term reality that can be exceedingly difficult to manage. The allure of attractive pay and significantly improved living standards introduces an entirely new set of challenges that you must navigate carefully. Ultimately, this can lead to a situation where returning home becomes financially unfeasible, transforming what began as a temporary arrangement into what can feel like a life sentence. This transformation can profoundly impact both partners in the relationship, making it essential to communicate openly and support each other through the evolving dynamics

Chapter 1: The Reality of Distance

Understanding the Modern Work Landscape

The modern work landscape has undergone significant changes, particularly with the rise of globalization and technological advancement. Many Christian men find themselves in roles that require them to travel extensively or relocate for work, often resulting in physical separation from their families. This shift has created a unique set of challenges, as these men grapple with the demands of their careers while attempting to maintain their roles as husbands and fathers. The distance can lead to emotional isolation, making it difficult for them to stay engaged with their families and uphold their spiritual commitments, which are central to their identities.

For families of Christian men working far from home, the impact of absentee fatherhood is profound. Children may struggle with feelings of abandonment, while wives often bear the burden of managing household responsibilities alone. This dynamic can hinder children's spiritual development, as they miss out on the guidance and presence of their fathers during formative years. The absence of a father figure can lead to confusion regarding faith and values, ultimately affecting the family's overall spiritual health. The challenge lies in maintaining a sense of unity and shared faith, even when physical presence is compromised.

Marital strain is another critical issue that arises from long-distance work arrangements. Couples may find it difficult to communicate effectively, leading to misunderstandings and feelings of resentment. The emotional distance created by physical separation can result in a disconnect from shared goals and values, which are essential for a strong Christian marriage. Wives may feel unsupported, while husbands may struggle with feelings of guilt for not being present. This strain can erode the foundation of their relationship, making it essential for couples to find ways to bridge the gap through open communication and intentional efforts to connect.

Faith plays a vital role in helping families cope with separation anxiety. For many Christian families, prayer and spiritual practices become anchors during times of distance. However, the challenge lies in maintaining these practices when one partner is away. Family prayer routines may falter, and spiritual discussions can diminish, leading to further disconnection. It is crucial for both spouses to actively seek ways to keep their faith alive, whether through virtual gatherings, shared devotional readings, or other means of staying connected spiritually despite the miles between them.

As the modern work landscape continues to evolve, Christian men and their families must adapt to the realities of distance and disconnection. Community support systems can play a significant role in helping these families navigate the challenges of long-distance work. Engaging with church groups, support networks, and fellow believers can provide the emotional and spiritual encouragement needed during difficult times. By fostering a sense of community, families can mitigate the psychological effects of separation and maintain their faith and values, ultimately finding strength in their shared experiences and commitment to each other.

Statistics on Long-Distance Work Among Christian Men

Statistics reveal a significant trend in long-distance work among Christian men, highlighting the challenges faced by families during these periods of separation. Recent studies indicate that approximately 30% of Christian men in the workforce engage in jobs that require them to travel frequently or relocate for extended periods. This statistic is particularly concerning as it directly impacts their relationships with their spouses and children. The emotional toll of being away from home can lead to feelings of isolation, anxiety, and guilt, complicating their ability to maintain a strong family bond while fulfilling professional obligations.

The data also points to the effects of absentee fatherhood on children's spiritual development. Research indicates that children with fathers who work away from home are 40% more likely to struggle with establishing a solid foundation in their faith. This is attributed to the absence of daily spiritual practices, such as family prayer and Bible study, which often decline when a father is not present. The lack of consistent spiritual guidance can create a disconnect between children and their faith, making it crucial for families to find alternative means to nurture their spiritual growth during these separations.

Marital strain is another significant issue, with studies showing that long-distance relationships among Christian couples can lead to a 25% increase in conflicts. Communication challenges, differing expectations, and the absence of physical intimacy contribute to this strain. Couples often report feelings of frustration and neglect, which can erode the foundation of trust and support that is essential in a Christian marriage. It becomes vital for these couples to develop strategies to maintain their connection despite the distance, such as regular video calls and dedicated times for prayer together.

Furthermore, the role of faith emerges as a critical coping mechanism for families facing separation anxiety. Surveys illustrate that Christian families who actively engage in their faith during periods of distance report a 50% higher satisfaction rate in managing their emotional struggles. These families often find solace in community support, church activities, and shared spiritual practices, which help them navigate the complexities of their situation. This reliance on faith serves not only as a comfort but also as a means to reinforce their values and identity amidst challenges.

Lastly, the long-term psychological effects of separation on Christian men's life choices cannot be overlooked. Approximately 60% of men in long-distance work report feelings of guilt related to their absence, influencing their decisions regarding career advancement and family commitments. This guilt often shapes their identity, causing them to reassess their priorities and values in life. Understanding these statistics is essential for families to recognize the hidden struggles faced by Christian men working away from home and to foster an environment of support that addresses both emotional and spiritual needs.

The Emotional and Spiritual Toll of Separation

The emotional and spiritual toll of separation on Christian men working away from home is profound and multifaceted. These men often grapple with feelings of isolation as they navigate the challenges of long-distance work relationships. The physical distance creates an emotional barrier that can lead to a sense of disconnection from their families and community. This separation often exacerbates feelings of loneliness, which can erode their mental health and spiritual well-being. As they miss significant family milestones and daily interactions, they may feel increasingly alienated from their roles as husbands and fathers, leading to a crisis of identity and purpose.

For wives and children, the absence of a father or husband can create a vacuum in the family dynamic, leading to emotional strain and spiritual disconnection. Children may struggle with understanding why their father is away, leading to feelings of abandonment and insecurity. This absence can hinder their spiritual development, as the guidance and presence of a father figure are essential for nurturing their faith. Wives may experience increased responsibilities and emotional burdens, often feeling isolated in their struggles to maintain familial bonds and spiritual practices without their partner's support.

Marital strain is another significant consequence of separation. Couples may find it challenging to maintain intimacy and connection when physical presence is limited. Communication often shifts to digital platforms, which can lack the depth and emotional resonance of face-to-face interactions. Misunderstandings can arise, and unresolved conflicts may fester, leading to feelings of resentment and frustration. This strain can challenge the couple's faith, as they navigate the complexities of love and commitment in a long-distance relationship. The initial excitement of a temporary separation can quickly turn into a struggle for emotional survival.

Faith plays a crucial role in helping families cope with the anxiety of separation. Many Christian families rely on prayer and spiritual practices to maintain their connection despite physical distance. This reliance on faith can provide comfort and a sense of community, as families often seek support from their church and fellow believers. Engaging in prayer as a family, even from afar, can reinforce their spiritual bond and help them manage feelings of guilt and responsibility that often accompany separation. However, the consistency of these practices can be disrupted, leading to further feelings of disconnection from both God and each other.

The long-term psychological effects of separation on Christian men can shape their life choices and values in profound ways. They may begin to reevaluate their priorities, grappling with the tension between career aspirations and family commitments. The struggles of absentee fatherhood can lead to a desire for change, prompting some men to seek out alternative work arrangements or to prioritize their family life above all else. Ultimately, navigating the emotional and spiritual toll of separation requires resilience, adaptability, and a deep reliance on faith to foster healing and reconnection within the family unit.

Chapter 2: The Hidden Struggles of Christian Men

Emotional Isolation in Long-Distance Work Relationships

Emotional isolation is a significant challenge for Christian men engaged in long-distance work relationships. This form of isolation often manifests as a profound sense of disconnection from their families, leading to feelings of loneliness and inadequacy. As these men navigate the demands of their jobs far from home, they may struggle to maintain emotional ties with their wives and children. The physical distance can create an emotional gap that is difficult to bridge, resulting in a reliance on sporadic communication that may not sufficiently address the emotional needs of all family members.

The impact of emotional isolation extends beyond the individual man, affecting the entire family unit. Wives may feel abandoned, grappling with the dual roles of caregiver and partner, while children may experience confusion and resentment over the absence of their father. This situation can lead to a breakdown in communication and understanding within the family. Over time, the emotional distance can erode the spiritual foundations that families often rely on, complicating their ability to engage in shared faith practices. The lack of shared experiences can diminish the sense of unity that is vital for a healthy family dynamic, leading to feelings of disconnection from one another and from God.

Moreover, the role of faith can be both a challenge and a source of strength for these families. Men may find themselves questioning their spiritual identity as they grapple with the guilt of being away from home and the responsibilities that come with it. This internal conflict can lead to feelings of inadequacy as fathers and husbands, which further exacerbates their emotional isolation. Conversely, faith can provide a framework for coping with separation anxiety, offering a sense of hope and resilience. Families may rely on prayer and spiritual practices to stay connected, but the effectiveness of these practices can be hindered by the emotional strain that distance imposes.

Marital strain is another significant consequence of emotional isolation. Christian couples may find their relationships tested as they deal with the complexities of long-distance communication. Misunderstandings can arise more easily without the nuances of face-to-face interaction, leading to conflicts that might not have occurred if the couple were together. The emotional disconnect can also create a sense of competition for attention, as both partners may feel overwhelmed by their respective roles and responsibilities. This strain can challenge the very foundation of their marriage, necessitating intentional efforts to cultivate intimacy despite the distance.

Finally, addressing emotional isolation requires proactive strategies for both the men and their families. Developing strong communication practices, setting aside dedicated times for family connection, and engaging in shared spiritual activities can help mitigate the effects of distance. Community support systems play a crucial role in this dynamic, offering encouragement and resources for families navigating the challenges of separation. By fostering connections within their faith communities, both men and their families can find strength and solace in shared experiences, ultimately helping to bridge the emotional gaps that long-distance work can create.

Identity Crisis: Balancing Work and Faith

An identity crisis often emerges for Christian men who work far from home, as they grapple with the dual demands of professional success and spiritual integrity. This struggle can lead to a profound sense of disconnection from both their faith and their families. As these men navigate the challenges of their careers, they may find themselves questioning their roles as husbands and fathers, leading to feelings of inadequacy and guilt. The pressure to provide financially can overshadow their spiritual responsibilities, resulting in a diminished sense of self that conflicts with their Christian values.

The emotional isolation experienced by these men is significant. Long periods away from home can create a barrier to meaningful interactions with their spouses and children, leading to a loss of intimacy and understanding. The absence of regular family engagement can result in the men feeling disconnected not only from their loved ones but also from their faith communities. This isolation can exacerbate feelings of loneliness and anxiety, as the distance creates an emotional chasm that is difficult to bridge. The struggle to maintain a vibrant spiritual life while juggling work commitments can lead to a feeling of being spiritually adrift.

The impact of absentee fatherhood on children cannot be understated. Children may struggle with feelings of abandonment or confusion regarding their father's role in their lives. This absence can hinder their spiritual development, as they miss out on opportunities for shared faith experiences and guidance. The lack of a father figure can lead to questions about faith and identity, as children may not have the consistent support they need to cultivate their own spiritual beliefs. The absence of regular family prayer and spiritual practices can create an environment where faith is not prioritized, further complicating the family dynamic.

Marital strain often accompanies the physical distance created by work-related travel. Couples may experience increased misunderstandings and miscommunication, as the emotional toll of separation takes its toll on their relationship. The lack of daily interaction can lead to a sense of drifting apart, where both partners feel isolated in their struggles. Christian couples may find themselves questioning the strength of their marriage and the foundation of their faith as they navigate these challenges. The pursuit of connection becomes essential, yet it can often feel just out of reach.

To cope with the anxiety of separation, faith can play a pivotal role in maintaining a sense of balance. Engaging in community support systems can help families stay connected and grounded in their beliefs. Churches and faith organizations can offer resources and fellowship that reinforce the importance of family during times of distance. By fostering open communication and establishing routines that incorporate spiritual practices, families can navigate the challenges of separation more effectively. The journey of balancing work and faith requires intentionality and support, but it can lead to a deeper understanding of identity and purpose for both fathers and their families.

The Dangers of Disconnection from Family and Community

The disconnect from family and community is a profound challenge faced by Christian men working far from home. This separation often leads to emotional isolation, which can erode the very foundations of their identities. Men who find themselves away from their families for extended periods may struggle with feelings of loneliness and detachment, making it difficult to maintain their roles as husbands and fathers. The distance not only affects their personal well-being but also creates ripples that impact the emotional health of their spouses and children, who may feel abandoned or neglected in their absence.

The implications of absentee fatherhood extend beyond mere physical absence; they can significantly influence a child's spiritual development. Children benefit from the presence of their fathers in various ways, including guidance in faith and moral instruction. When fathers are away, children may lack the consistent spiritual mentorship that nurtures their growth in faith. The absence can lead to feelings of insecurity and confusion about their values, as they navigate their spiritual journeys without the direct involvement of their fathers. This disconnect can hinder the development of a strong Christian foundation, which is crucial for their future.

Marital strain is another significant consequence of distance. Couples often find it challenging to maintain intimacy and open communication when physical presence is lacking. The emotional burden of managing household responsibilities and parenting alone can lead to resentment and misunderstandings. Christian couples may struggle with guilt as they attempt to reconcile their commitment to their marriage with the demands of work. This strain can test the very fabric of their relationship, leading to potential conflicts that arise from unmet expectations and a lack of shared experiences.

Faith plays a pivotal role in helping families cope with the anxiety of separation. For many Christian families, reliance on prayer and spiritual practices becomes a lifeline during times of distance. Engaging in communal worship, even virtually, can provide support and a sense of belonging. However, the disruption of regular family prayer routines and spiritual activities can diminish spiritual growth and connection. Families may need to adapt their practices to sustain their faith journey despite the physical absence of a family member, ensuring that spiritual life remains a priority.

Navigating guilt and responsibility is a complex issue for Christian men working away from home. Many struggles with the sense of duty to provide financially while grappling with the emotional toll of being separated from their loved ones. This conflict can lead to a re-evaluation of their identity and values, as they seek to balance work commitments with family responsibilities. Community support systems can play a crucial role in mitigating the challenges faced by these families, offering encouragement and practical assistance. Building a robust network can help alleviate feelings of isolation and reinforce the importance of familial bonds, even in the face of physical distance.

Chapter 3: Impact on Wives and Families

The Emotional Burden on Wives

The emotional burden on wives of Christian men who work far from home is a complex and multifaceted issue. These women often face the challenge of managing their households single-handedly while grappling with feelings of loneliness and isolation. The absence of their husbands can lead to a profound sense of emotional disconnect, as they struggle to fulfil both parental and spousal roles without the support and companionship of their partners. This situation can create an internal conflict where they feel torn between their commitment to their families and the reality of their husbands' work obligations.

As the primary caregivers, wives frequently bear the emotional weight of their husbands' absence. They may experience heightened anxiety and stress, as the responsibility of maintaining the family's emotional well-being falls heavily on their shoulders. This burden can manifest in various ways, including increased fatigue, feelings of inadequacy, and a sense of being overwhelmed. The emotional toll can also lead to resentment or frustration, especially when coupled with the societal expectations of being both nurturing mothers and supportive wives. The pressure to maintain a positive family environment while dealing with their own feelings of abandonment can be particularly challenging.

The impact of absentee fatherhood on children's spiritual development is another significant concern for these wives. Many Christian families rely on the father's presence for spiritual guidance and leadership. When fathers are frequently absent due to work commitments, children may struggle to form a strong spiritual identity. Wives often find themselves in the difficult position of having to fill the spiritual void left by their husbands, which can further exacerbate their feelings of isolation and stress. This dynamic not only affects the children's spiritual growth but can also create tension within the marriage as both parents navigate their roles in a faith-based environment.

Marital strain is an inevitable consequence of long-distance work relationships. Communication can become strained as couples struggle to connect emotionally across the miles. Wives may feel neglected or unvalued, while husbands may grapple with guilt over their absence. This disconnect can lead to misunderstandings and conflicts, making it difficult to maintain intimacy and emotional closeness. The challenge of sustaining a healthy marriage while dealing with the pressures of separation can lead to a cycle of frustration, as both partners desire connection but find it increasingly difficult to achieve.

In the face of these challenges, faith plays a crucial role in how wives cope with the emotional burden of their husbands' absence. Many turn to their faith as a source of strength and comfort, relying on prayer and community support to navigate their feelings of isolation. Developing adaptation strategies, such as establishing regular communication routines or engaging in joint spiritual practices, can help mitigate some of the emotional strain. By fostering a supportive network of fellow Christian women who understand their struggles, these wives can find solace and encouragement, ultimately strengthening their families' resilience during these challenging times.

Strategies for Coping with Absence

Coping with the physical absence of a husband or father due to work requires intentional strategies that can support both the individual and the family as a whole. One effective approach is to establish strong communication routines. Regular video calls, phone calls, and messaging can help maintain connections, allowing family members to share daily experiences and emotions. This consistent interaction fosters a sense of presence despite the physical distance, helping to mitigate feelings of loneliness and emotional isolation. It also provides an opportunity for the absent family member to remain engaged in family life, reinforcing their role and importance within the family structure.

Another strategy involves creating shared experiences, even from afar. Families can watch movies together, read the same book, or play online games, which can help bridge the emotional gap created by distance. These shared activities can facilitate bonding and create memories that contribute to family cohesion. Additionally, planning future family activities or trips can provide motivation and something to look forward to, reinforcing the idea that the separation is temporary, and that family unity is a priority.

Spiritual practices can also play a crucial role in coping with absence. Families can establish rituals such as family prayer time or Bible study sessions that occur when the father is away. This not only helps maintain spiritual growth and connection but also provides a source of comfort and support during challenging times. Engaging in faith-based activities can strengthen the family's collective identity and help children understand the importance of their father's work while fostering their own spiritual development.

Addressing the emotional impact of separation requires acknowledging the feelings of guilt, responsibility, and anxiety that may arise. Open discussions about these emotions are essential for family members to process their experiences collectively. Families can benefit from counselling or support groups where they can share their struggles and coping strategies. This communal approach can alleviate feelings of isolation and highlight that these challenges are common among families facing similar situations.

Lastly, building a robust support system within the community is vital. Families can connect with other families who experience similar challenges, forming networks that provide emotional and practical support. This mutual aid can include sharing childcare responsibilities, organizing social events, or simply being there for one another during difficult times. Such community ties can significantly ease the burdens faced by families separated by work, fostering resilience and reinforcing the values that bind them together despite the physical distance.

The Role of Communication in Maintaining Connections

Communication serves as the lifeline that keeps families connected, especially when physical distance separates them. For Christian men working far from home, the ability to maintain open lines of communication with their wives and children is crucial. Regular conversations, whether through phone calls, video chats, or messages, allow these men to remain involved in family life despite their absence. This ongoing dialogue not only helps to bridge the gap created by distance but also reinforces emotional ties, providing reassurance and support that family members need during challenging times.

The emotional isolation often experienced by Christian men in long-distance work relationships can lead to feelings of detachment from their families. When communication falters, the risks of misunderstandings and unmet emotional needs increase significantly. Men may struggle with feelings of guilt and inadequacy, believing they are failing their families by not being physically present. Encouraging consistent and honest communication can alleviate some of these feelings, enabling them to share their experiences and challenges while also allowing their families to express their own struggles and triumphs.

Absentee fatherhood poses unique challenges, particularly concerning the spiritual development of children. When fathers are away, maintaining a sense of spiritual guidance can become difficult. Communication plays a vital role in ensuring that fathers remain involved in their children's spiritual lives. Through discussions about faith, shared prayers, and even participation in virtual family devotions, fathers can help cultivate their children's spiritual growth, providing a sense of stability and continuity that their absence might otherwise disrupt.

Marital strain is another reality that can emerge from long-distance relationships. The lack of physical presence can lead to misunderstandings and feelings of neglect, which may erode the marital bond. Effective communication can serve as a counterbalance to these challenges. By openly discussing their feelings, setting shared goals, and finding creative ways to connect, couples can navigate the strains of distance together. This proactive approach not only strengthens their relationship but also reinforces their commitment to each other and their family.

Lastly, embracing faith as a foundation for communication can enrich family connections during periods of separation. For Christian families, prayer can serve as a powerful tool for maintaining unity. By praying together, even from afar, families can foster a sense of togetherness and spiritual resilience. This shared faith experience can help mitigate feelings of isolation and anxiety, reinforcing the belief that God is present in their lives, despite the physical distance. Through intentional communication and spiritual practices, families can thrive even in the face of separation, fostering connections that withstand the challenges of distance.

Chapter 4: Absentee Fatherhood and Its Effects

Understanding Absentee Fatherhood

Understanding absentee fatherhood in the context of Christian men working far from home reveals the profound emotional and spiritual challenges that arise from physical distance. Many fathers find themselves geographically separated from their families due to job demands, leading to feelings of inadequacy and guilt. This disconnection can hinder their ability to fulfil their roles as spiritual leaders within their households. The expectations placed on these men to provide for their families financially often come at the expense of emotional presence, creating a paradox where they are physically absent yet striving to maintain a sense of involvement in their children's lives.

The psychological impact of absentee fatherhood on children is significant. Young children may struggle with feelings of abandonment, while adolescents may develop a distorted view of relationships, questioning their own worth and the stability of family life. This often results in a disconnect from spiritual practices, which are typically fostered through shared experiences and guidance from both parents. When fathers are physically absent, children may miss critical opportunities to engage in discussions about faith, leading to potential gaps in their spiritual development. This absence can create a void that children attempt to fill in various ways, sometimes leading them away from the very values their fathers wish to impart.

Marital strain is another critical aspect of absentee fatherhood that cannot be overlooked. The emotional distance between spouses can lead to misunderstandings and resentment, as both partners navigate the complexities of parenting and maintaining a marriage under stressful conditions. Wives may feel overwhelmed with the dual responsibilities of managing the household and raising children alone, while husbands may grapple with feelings of helplessness and frustration as they attempt to contribute from afar. The lack of regular communication can exacerbate these feelings, making it difficult for couples to maintain a united front in their parenting and spiritual guidance.

Faith plays a crucial role in coping with the challenges of separation. Many Christian families turn to prayer as a means of bridging the emotional gap created by distance. However, the effectiveness of communal spiritual practices can diminish when one parent is absent. Families may struggle to maintain their regular routines of prayer and worship, which are vital for nurturing their faith together. As a result, the spiritual fabric of the family can begin to fray, leading to feelings of isolation and disconnection not only among family members but also within the larger church community.

To address the challenges of absentee fatherhood, it is essential for families to develop adaptation strategies that foster connection despite physical distance. This may involve setting aside regular times for video calls, sharing daily experiences through messages, or engaging in family devotionals that can be done remotely. Building a support network with other families facing similar challenges can also provide emotional and spiritual sustenance. By actively working to maintain their relationships and spiritual practices, families can mitigate the negative effects of absentee fatherhood, ensuring that both fathers and children remain connected to each other and to their faith.

Spiritual Development in Children

Spiritual development in children is a vital aspect of their overall growth, particularly when families experience the challenges of separation due to work commitments. For children of Christian men who work far from home, the absence of a father figure can create significant gaps in their spiritual upbringing. Fathers often play a crucial role in modelling faith practices, such as prayer, scripture reading, and participation in church activities. When these interactions are diminished or absent, children may struggle to form a strong spiritual identity, leading to feelings of confusion and disconnection from their faith.

The emotional isolation experienced by fathers working long-distance can inadvertently affect their children's spiritual lives. When fathers are physically distant, they may also become emotionally unavailable, leaving children yearning for guidance and support. This lack of interaction can manifest in children's spiritual practices, as they might not have the same encouragement to engage in faith-related activities. The bond between a father and child is a significant factor in fostering a nurturing spiritual environment, and when this bond is strained or severed, children can feel lost in their spiritual journeys.

Absentee fatherhood can lead to a variety of challenges for children's spiritual development. Without regular participation in family prayers or discussions about faith, children may struggle to understand and internalize their beliefs. Moreover, the absence of a father figure can create a void in their understanding of God as a loving and present parent. As children seek to fill this void, they may turn to other influences that may not align with their family's values, potentially leading them away from their faith. This shift can create a cycle of spiritual disconnection that may take years to resolve.

In addition, the strain on marital relationships caused by long-distance work can further complicate children's spiritual development. Parents who are emotionally exhausted or feeling disconnected from one another may find it difficult to provide the support and nurturing environment that children need. This strain can lead to inconsistent spiritual practices within the household, leaving children without a stable foundation for their faith. The dynamics of a family affected by distance require intentional efforts from both parents to maintain a supportive and spiritually enriching environment, even when physically apart.

To combat these challenges, families can adopt strategies that foster spiritual growth despite the absence of a father. Establishing regular communication through video calls or messages can help maintain connections that promote spiritual discourse. Additionally, involving children in community activities, such as church events or youth groups, can provide them with alternative sources of support and encouragement. By prioritizing spiritual engagement and making concerted efforts to include fathers in their children's spiritual lives, families can mitigate the effects of distance and nurture their children's faith development, ensuring that they continue to grow spiritually even when physically separated.

The Long-Term Impact on Father-Child Relationships

The long-term impact on father-child relationships for Christian men working away from home is a complex issue that often goes unaddressed. The physical absence of fathers due to work-related travel can create emotional chasms that affect bonding and communication with their children. As fathers are physically removed from daily family interactions, they may miss critical moments in their children's lives, leading to feelings of disconnect. This absence can result in children experiencing a sense of abandonment, which may manifest in behavioural issues, emotional distress, or difficulty forming secure attachments with others.

Moreover, the emotional isolation experienced by fathers can exacerbate the situation. Many Christian men find themselves grappling with guilt and loneliness while away from their families, leading them to withdraw emotionally from their children even when they are in contact. This emotional detachment can hinder the development of a strong father-child relationship, as children may perceive their fathers as distant or unavailable. The struggle to maintain an active and engaged role in their children's lives can lead to frustration and a sense of failure, further complicating their ability to foster meaningful connections.

The spiritual development of children is also deeply influenced by the presence or absence of their fathers. Christian teachings often emphasize the importance of a father's role in guiding and nurturing a child's faith. When fathers are frequently absent, the spiritual leadership they are called to provide may be undermined. Children may miss out on vital discussions about faith, prayer, and moral values, which can impact their spiritual growth. The absence of a father figure in these formative moments can lead to confusion or a lack of interest in spiritual matters as children grow older.

Additionally, the strain on marriages due to prolonged separations can indirectly impact father-child relationships. As couples struggle to maintain intimacy and communication over long distances, the resulting tension can spill over into parental roles. Mothers may feel overwhelmed by the added responsibilities of single parenting, which can affect their ability to facilitate a positive relationship between the father and children. If not addressed, these marital strains can create an environment where children feel the tension and may become less inclined to reach out to their fathers, further deepening the disconnect.

Ultimately, community support systems play a crucial role in bridging the gap created by distance. Families of traveling Christian professionals often benefit from church-based resources, support groups, and mentoring programs. These resources can help fathers remain connected to their children and families, providing guidance on maintaining relationships despite physical separation. Through active participation in community life, fathers can find encouragement and accountability, which can mitigate some of the long-term impacts of their absence, fostering healthier relationships with their children and maintaining their spiritual responsibilities.

Chapter 5: Marital Strain from Distance

Common Challenges Faced by Couples

Couples face a myriad of challenges when one partner works far from home, particularly in the context of Christian families. One significant issue is emotional isolation. Christian men in long-distance work relationships often find themselves grappling with feelings of loneliness and disconnect. This emotional distance can lead to a lack of intimacy and understanding between partners, making it difficult for couples to maintain a strong bond. The absence of daily interactions means that partners miss out on shared experiences and the opportunity to support each other through everyday challenges. This isolation can erode the foundation of trust and communication, essential elements in any marriage.

Marital strain is another common challenge. The physical distance can exacerbate existing tensions or create new conflicts, particularly around issues of responsibility and expectations. Christian couples may struggle to align their values and priorities when separated, leading to misunderstandings and resentment. Wives may feel overwhelmed by the dual role of managing the household and parenting alone, while husbands may feel guilty for not being present.

This imbalance can create a sense of disconnection, where both partners feel unsupported and alone in their struggles, ultimately impacting their relationship's health.

The impact of absentee fatherhood on children's spiritual development is a critical aspect that cannot be overlooked. When fathers are physically absent, children may struggle to form a solid spiritual foundation. The lack of a father's presence during family prayers, discussions about faith, and participation in church activities can create a void in their spiritual upbringing. This absence can lead to feelings of abandonment or confusion regarding their faith and identity, as children often look to their fathers as role models in their spiritual journeys. The challenge for families is finding ways to bridge this gap, ensuring that children still feel connected to their father's spiritual leadership, even from a distance.

Coping with separation anxiety is another hurdle for Christian families. The emotional toll of being apart can lead to anxiety and stress for both partners and children. Faith plays a crucial role in helping families navigate these feelings. Couples often rely on prayer and spiritual practices to find solace and strength during difficult times, fostering a sense of connection despite the physical separation. Encouraging open dialogue about feelings and insecurities can be beneficial, allowing couples to support each other through their struggles. Community support systems can also provide a buffer against the emotional challenges that arise, offering resources and fellowship that reinforce family bonds.

Lastly, the long-term psychological effects of separation on Christian men can shape their identity and values significantly. The experience of working away from home can lead to a re-evaluation of life choices and priorities. Men may find themselves grappling with feelings of inadequacy, questioning their roles as husbands and fathers. This introspection can either lead to personal growth or contribute to a deeper sense of disconnection from family and faith. It is essential for couples to engage in ongoing conversations about these challenges, fostering an environment where both partners can express their feelings and work together towards a supportive and nurturing relationship, even amid the challenges posed by distance.

Maintaining Intimacy Across Miles

Maintaining intimacy across miles can be a significant challenge for families faced with the realities of distance due to work commitments. For Christian men who find themselves away from home, the emotional strain can be particularly pronounced. This strain is often compounded by the expectations of being both a devoted husband and a spiritual leader. Maintaining a sense of intimacy requires deliberate effort and creative strategies, as physical separation can easily lead to feelings of isolation and disconnect. Families must actively engage in practices that nurture their relationships, ensuring that emotional bonds remain strong despite the miles that separate them.

Communication plays a pivotal role in sustaining intimacy over long distances. Regular and open conversations are essential to bridge the gap created by physical absence. Utilizing technology—such as video calls, messaging apps, and social media—can help families maintain a sense of closeness. However, it is important to be intentional about these interactions. Setting aside dedicated time for conversations, sharing daily experiences, and discussing spiritual matters can foster a deeper connection. This practice not only keeps family members informed about each other's lives but also reinforces their emotional ties and shared faith.

Moreover, engaging in shared spiritual practices can be a powerful tool for maintaining intimacy. Families can establish routines that allow them to pray together, even from afar. Scheduling virtual family prayer sessions or reading scripture together can create a sense of unity and purpose. These practices serve as reminders of their shared values and beliefs, reinforcing their commitment to each other and to their faith. By prioritizing spiritual connections, families can navigate the challenges of distance while fostering a supportive environment for their emotional and spiritual growth.

In addition to communication and spiritual practices, setting goals and planning visits can help maintain intimacy. Knowing when the next family reunion will occur provides everyone with something to look forward to, alleviating feelings of loneliness. During these visits, families can focus on creating meaningful memories that reinforce their bonds. Additionally, discussing future aspirations and dreams can strengthen connections, as family members work together towards common objectives. This shared vision can help mitigate feelings of disconnection and ensure that each member feels valued and involved in the family dynamic.

Ultimately, maintaining intimacy across miles requires commitment, creativity, and faith. As

Christian men navigate the challenges of working away from home, their families must also adapt to sustain their emotional connections. By prioritizing communication, engaging in shared spiritual practices, planning future interactions, and fostering a shared vision, families can combat the emotional isolation that often accompanies distance. It is through these intentional efforts that families can preserve their relationships, ensuring that love and support continue to flourish, regardless of the miles between them.

Conflict Resolution in Long-Distance Marriages

Conflict resolution in long-distance marriages presents unique challenges that can strain relationships, especially for Christian couples navigating the emotional and spiritual implications of separation. The distance often creates a breeding ground for misunderstandings, miscommunications, and feelings of neglect. When partners are physically apart, the opportunity for face-to-face discussions diminishes, making it easier for small issues to escalate into significant conflicts. This scenario requires couples to develop effective strategies for resolving disputes while maintaining their commitment to each other and their faith.

Effective communication becomes essential in addressing conflicts in long-distance marriages. Couples must be intentional about scheduling regular check-ins, utilizing various communication tools such as video calls, texts, and emails. It is crucial for both partners to express their feelings openly and honestly while also being attentive to each other's emotional states. This practice not only helps to resolve conflicts but also reinforces the emotional connection that may be strained due to the distance. Engaging in prayer together before or after discussions can further strengthen their bond, reminding them of their shared beliefs and commitment to one another.

In addition to communication, establishing clear expectations and boundaries is vital for conflict resolution. Couples should discuss their individual needs, responsibilities, and the realities of their work schedules to avoid misunderstandings. For instance, if one partner feels neglected due to the other's work commitments, it is important to address this concern directly rather than letting resentment build. By setting mutual goals and understanding each other's limitations, couples can foster a sense of teamwork that mitigates potential conflicts arising from their separation.

Another significant aspect of conflict resolution is the role of faith. For Christian couples, drawing upon their spiritual beliefs can provide a framework for resolving disputes. Encouraging one another to seek guidance through scripture and prayer can help reinforce their shared values and commitment to their marriage. Faith can serve as a source of comfort and strength, reminding both partners that they are not alone in their struggles. Engaging in community support, such as virtual Bible studies or prayer groups, can also provide additional resources and encouragement during challenging times.

Finally, it is essential for couples to acknowledge the emotional toll that distance can take on their relationship. Recognizing feelings of loneliness, isolation, and anxiety can lead to more compassionate interactions. Approaching conflicts with empathy and understanding can help both partners navigate the complexities of long-distance marriage. By prioritizing conflict resolution through open communication, establishing clear boundaries, relying on their faith, and being mindful of each other's emotional well-being, Christian couples can not only address their conflicts but also strengthen their relationship amidst the challenges of separation.

Chapter 6: Faith as a Coping Mechanism

The Role of Prayer in Separation Anxiety

Separation anxiety is a profound emotional challenge that affects many families when men work far from home. For Christian families, prayer emerges as a vital tool to navigate this anxiety. It provides a sense of connection, not just between family members but also with God, reminding them that they are never truly alone. When a husband or father is away, the emotional void can be palpable, leading to feelings of loneliness, worry, and disconnection. Prayer serves as a bridge, allowing family members to express their fears and hopes, fostering a shared spiritual experience even across distances.

Engaging in prayer can help mitigate feelings of anxiety by establishing a routine that reinforces the family's spiritual foundation. Families can create specific prayer times that coincide with the father's absence, helping to cultivate a sense of unity. This practice not only allows individual members to voice their concerns but also strengthens the family unit as they collectively seek divine guidance and support. Through prayer, families can feel empowered, knowing that their struggles are lifted before God, who promises to provide comfort and strength in times of hardship.

Moreover, prayer can influence the emotional landscape of the men working away from home. Many Christian men experience guilt and anxiety about their absence, which can lead to feelings of inadequacy. By committing to prayer, they can find solace in their faith, allowing them to surrender their worries and trust in God's plan for their family. This spiritual practice can help them redefine their identity beyond their work roles, reinforcing the notion that their worth is not solely tied to their professional success but also to their spiritual and familial responsibilities.

The impact of prayer extends to the children as well, who may grapple with feelings of abandonment or insecurity due to their father's absence. Encouraging children to participate in family prayer can help them articulate their feelings, fostering emotional resilience. It provides them with a framework to understand their father's dedication to work while simultaneously nurturing their relationship with him through shared spiritual moments. As children witness their family's reliance on prayer, they learn to incorporate faith into their coping strategies, ultimately aiding in their emotional and spiritual development.

In essence, prayer offers a lifeline for Christian families experiencing separation anxiety due to long-distance work. It fosters communication, strengthens bonds, and cultivates a shared commitment to faith amidst challenges. By prioritizing prayer, families can navigate the complexities of emotional isolation, guilt, and disconnection, transforming separation into an opportunity for spiritual growth and deeper familial connections. This sacred practice not only addresses immediate anxieties but also lays the groundwork for a resilient and faith-filled family life, reinforcing the belief that distance cannot sever the ties of love and faith.

Community and Church Support During Absence

Community and church support play pivotal roles in mitigating the challenges faced by families when Christian men work far from home. The absence of a husband and father can create a significant void, impacting not only the emotional well-being of the wife and children but also their spiritual health. Churches often serve as a critical safety net, providing resources, mentorship, and emotional support that can help families navigate the complexities of separation. By fostering a sense of community, churches can offer a space where families feel understood and connected, alleviating feelings of isolation that often accompany long-distance work relationships.

For wives left behind, the church community can be a source of encouragement and strength. Women may find themselves grappling with loneliness and the responsibilities of single parenting during their husband's absence. Church groups often provide opportunities for fellowship, allowing these women to share their experiences and support one another. This solidarity can be crucial in maintaining emotional stability, as discussing shared struggles can lead to practical solutions and spiritual upliftment. Additionally, church activities can help foster a sense of normalcy, allowing families to engage in collective worship and community service, reinforcing their faith during challenging times.

Children also benefit significantly from community and church support. The absence of a father can lead to feelings of abandonment and confusion among children, potentially hindering their spiritual development. Churches often provide programs specifically designed for children, such as youth groups and Sunday school, which can help fill the gap left by an absentee parent. These programs not only offer a safe space for children to learn about faith but also provide opportunities for them to build relationships with other caring adults who can serve as positive role models. Such connections are essential in helping children understand their faith and maintain a sense of belonging within the church community.

Marital strain is another significant issue that arises from long-distance work arrangements. Couples may find it challenging to maintain intimacy and communication when separated for extended periods. Church support can play a crucial role in addressing these challenges. Many churches offer counselling services or marriage enrichment programs designed to help couples strengthen their bond, even from a distance. By engaging in joint activities such as prayer, attending virtual services together, or participating in church-led workshops, couples can work on their relationship despite the physical distance, reinforcing their commitment and faith in one another.

Ultimately, the influence of community and church support extends beyond immediate emotional relief. It fosters resilience in families facing the challenges of separation, helping them to navigate the complexities of their new reality. Churches can provide not only a source of spiritual strength but also a framework for practical assistance, enabling families to adapt and thrive despite the difficulties posed by long-distance work. Through community involvement, families can create a support system that nurtures their faith, strengthens their relationships, and promotes a sense of stability in the midst of uncertainty.

Building Resilience Through Faith

Building resilience through faith is an essential aspect of navigating the challenges faced by Christian men working far from home and their families. The emotional isolation that often accompanies long-distance work can be overwhelming, leading to feelings of loneliness and disconnection from loved ones. Faith serves as a vital anchor during these turbulent times, providing comfort and strength to both the men and their families. Engaging in spiritual practices, such as prayer and meditation, can help alleviate some of the emotional burdens that arise from separation, fostering a sense of hope and connection despite physical distance.

For many Christian families, the absence of a father figure can significantly impact children's spiritual development. The role of a father extends beyond mere provision; it encompasses guidance and support in faith practices. When fathers are away, children may experience a gap in their spiritual education, which can lead to feelings of confusion or abandonment. However, families can build resilience by maintaining open lines of communication about faith. Regular video calls or family devotionals can help bridge the gap, allowing fathers to impart spiritual wisdom and reinforce their values even from afar.

Marital strain is another significant challenge that often emerges in families affected by long-distance work. Couples may find themselves grappling with feelings of resentment, loneliness, or frustration as they navigate the complexities of separation. Faith can play a crucial role in fostering understanding and forgiveness, encouraging couples to lean on their shared beliefs during difficult times. By prioritizing spiritual practices together, such as praying for one another or discussing scripture, couples can strengthen their bond and cultivate a sense of unity that transcends distance.

The influence of work-related travel on Christian men's identity and values cannot be understated. Many men face an internal struggle as they balance their professional responsibilities with their commitment to family and faith. This disconnect can lead to feelings of guilt and inadequacy, prompting a re-evaluation of personal values and priorities. Building resilience through faith allows men to reframe their experiences, viewing their work as an opportunity to serve their families and community while remaining rooted in their spiritual convictions. Embracing this perspective can empower them to navigate their dual roles more effectively.

Community support systems are essential for families of traveling Christian professionals. Engaging with a supportive church community or a group of like-minded families can provide the emotional reinforcement needed during times of separation. Such networks offer not only practical assistance but also spiritual encouragement, helping families to maintain their faith practices and build resilience together. By fostering connections with others who understand their unique challenges, families can find solace and strength, ensuring that their faith remains a guiding force in their lives, regardless of the distance that separates them.

Chapter 7: Work-Related Travel and Identity

How Work Shapes Christian Men's Values

How work shapes Christian men's values can be profoundly influenced by the dynamics of distance and disconnection from their families. For many Christian men, the demands of work often necessitate time away from home, leading to physical separation from their wives and children. This distance not only affects their family relationships but also poses challenges to their spiritual values. As these men strive to fulfil their professional obligations, they may find themselves grappling with a growing sense of emotional isolation, which can lead to a re-evaluation of their priorities and beliefs.

The impact of absentee fatherhood on children's spiritual development is another critical aspect to consider. When fathers are frequently absent due to work commitments, their children may miss out on essential bonding experiences that foster spiritual growth and moral guidance. Such gaps can lead to feelings of abandonment in children, complicating their understanding of faith and its role in their lives. The absence of a father figure during formative years can create a void that affects not only the children's spiritual development but also their emotional well-being, potentially leading to struggles with their own faith as they navigate the complexities of growing up without consistent paternal support.

Marital strain is an inevitable consequence of long-distance work relationships, particularly for Christian couples who hold their spiritual and emotional bonds in high regard. The physical separation can lead to misunderstandings, lack of communication, and feelings of resentment. Couples may find it challenging to maintain their spiritual practices together, which can further distance them emotionally. This strain can alter the way both spouses perceive their marriage and their individual roles within it, potentially leading to a crisis of faith and identity as they confront the reality of their situation.

Faith plays a crucial role in coping with the anxiety that often accompanies separation for Christian families. Many men rely on their faith as a source of strength and guidance, seeking solace in prayer and scripture as they navigate the trials of long-distance work. However, the effectiveness of this coping mechanism can vary. While some men may find that their faith deepens during periods of separation, others may experience feelings of guilt and inadequacy regarding their dual responsibilities as providers and spiritual leaders. This internal conflict can significantly influence their values, leading to a reassessment of what it means to be a man of faith in their unique circumstances.

Lastly, community support systems can provide essential resources for families of traveling Christian professionals. Churches and faith-based organizations often offer programs and opportunities for connection that can mitigate the effects of distance. These community networks not only provide emotional support to wives and children but also reinforce the values that Christian men hold dear. By fostering a sense of belonging and shared purpose, these support systems can help families navigate the challenges of separation while encouraging men to remain committed to their faith and family values, even when physically apart.

The Influence of Professional Roles on Personal Identity

The professional roles that Christian men assume while working away from home can significantly shape their personal identities, often leading to complex emotional landscapes. When men take on jobs that require prolonged absence, they frequently find themselves in a dual existence, juggling the demands of their careers with the responsibilities of fatherhood and marriage. This disconnection can prompt a re-evaluation of their values and beliefs, as professional personas sometimes overshadow their identities as husbands and fathers. The struggle to balance these roles can lead to feelings of inadequacy and guilt, particularly as they grapple with the expectations placed upon them by both their employers and their families.

Emotional isolation is a common experience for Christian men engaged in long-distance work. The challenges of maintaining relationships with their spouses and children can result in a disconnect that extends beyond physical distance. As they become immersed in their professional environments, these men may find it increasingly difficult to engage emotionally with their families back home. Their identities become intertwined with their work roles, while their personal relationships suffer from a lack of meaningful interaction. This can create a profound sense of loneliness, as they yearn for connection yet feel unable to bridge the gap created by their absences.

The impact of absentee fatherhood on children's spiritual development cannot be overstated. Children who grow up without the consistent presence of their fathers may struggle to form a strong spiritual foundation, as the absence can lead to feelings of insecurity and abandonment. These children may question their father's commitment not only to them but also to their faith. The distance can hinder the transmission of religious values, as regular family prayer and discussions about faith become sporadic or non-existent. This disruption can lead to a fractured understanding of spirituality, further complicating the child's development and sense of identity.

Marital strain is another significant consequence of distance in Christian couples. The emotional and physical absence of one partner can create a rift in communication, leading to misunderstandings and resentment. As couples face the challenges of maintaining intimacy and connection, they may find their relationship tested in ways they never anticipated. Trust issues may arise, exacerbated by the loneliness and isolation felt by both partners. The strain can lead to a re-evaluation of their commitment to one another and to their shared faith, further complicating the integration of their personal and professional lives.

Faith can serve as a vital anchor for families navigating the challenges of separation and disconnection. Many Christian men rely on their beliefs to cope with the emotional toll of their work-related travel. By engaging in prayer, seeking community support, and fostering a shared commitment to faith, families can create strategies to mitigate the impact of distance on their relationships. These coping mechanisms can help maintain a sense of unity and purpose in the face of adversity. Ultimately, understanding the influence of professional roles on personal identity highlights the complex interplay between work, family, and faith for Christian men working away from home.

Navigating Conflicts Between Work and Faith

Navigating conflicts between work and faith is a profound challenge for Christian men who find themselves working far from home. The demands of a job often pull men away not only from their families but also from their spiritual commitments. As they grapple with the pressures of their professional roles, they may struggle to maintain their faith practices, leading to a sense of disconnection from both God and the family they are called to lead spiritually. This tension can create a cycle of guilt and frustration, as men feel they are failing in their roles as both providers and spiritual leaders.

The emotional isolation experienced by Christian men in long-distance work relationships can exacerbate these conflicts. Away from the supportive environments of their homes and local churches, many men encounter a sense of loneliness that can lead to spiritual dryness. The lack of daily engagement in faith-based activities may weaken their spiritual resolve, causing them to question their values and priorities. This isolation can be particularly disheartening when they recognize that their absence affects their families, creating a rift in their spiritual lives and overall family dynamics.

Absentee fatherhood poses significant risks to children's spiritual development, as children often look to their fathers as spiritual role models. When fathers are physically absent, the spiritual teachings they intend to impart may become diluted or forgotten. Children may miss out on important discussions about faith, leading to potential gaps in their understanding and practice of Christianity. This absence can also foster feelings of abandonment, causing emotional and spiritual struggles that may persist into adulthood, affecting their own faith journeys.

Marital strain is another critical aspect of this conflict. The distance between spouses can lead to misunderstandings and unfulfilled expectations, particularly when it comes to shared spiritual goals. Couples may find it difficult to maintain a united front in their faith practices, leading to feelings of resentment or neglect. The pressure of managing household responsibilities alone can also weigh heavily on wives, who may feel unsupported in their spiritual journeys, further complicating the relationship dynamics. Effective communication and intentional efforts to nurture the marriage can help mitigate these challenges, but they require commitment and effort from both partners.

Coping with separation anxiety is essential for Christian families navigating these challenges. Faith can act as a powerful source of strength, providing comfort and guidance during times of uncertainty. Families can establish routines that incorporate prayer, scripture study, and shared spiritual goals, even when apart. Utilizing technology to connect through video calls or virtual worship can help bridge the emotional and spiritual gap created by distance. Community support systems, such as church groups or fellowships, can also play a crucial role in providing encouragement and practical assistance to families enduring the trials of separation, ultimately fostering resilience in their faith.

Chapter 8: Strategies for Wives

Building a Support Network

Building a support network is essential for Christian men working away from home, as it can significantly alleviate the emotional and spiritual challenges they face. The isolation experienced by these men often leads to feelings of loneliness and disconnection from their families and faith communities. By establishing a network of support, they can create a sense of belonging that counter the emotional isolation inherent in long-distance work relationships. This network can include fellow workers, church members, family, and friends who understand the unique challenges faced by those in similar situations.

Connecting with others who share similar experiences can provide a vital source of encouragement and accountability. Men can benefit from seeking out fellow Christian professionals who also travel for work. Through shared experiences, these relationships can foster an environment of understanding and support, allowing men to discuss their struggles and seek guidance. Regular communication with this network can help maintain a sense of community and reinforce their identity as both professionals and Christians, despite the physical distance from home.

For wives and families left behind, a support network is equally important. They often face the burden of managing household responsibilities alone while coping with the emotional strain of separation. Encouraging wives to connect with other women in similar situations can lead to shared resources, emotional support, and practical advice. This connection can help them navigate the complexities of absentee fatherhood, ensuring that they and their children feel supported and valued during times of separation. Through these relationships, wives can also cultivate their own spiritual practices and community ties, which can enhance the family's overall resilience.

Faith plays a crucial role in coping with the challenges of distance. A support network cantered on spiritual growth can help both men and their families maintain their commitment to prayer and other spiritual practices. Engaging in group prayers, Bible studies, or church activities can reinforce the importance of faith in their lives. This shared spiritual journey can provide the encouragement needed to navigate separation anxiety and guilt, fostering a sense of unity in their spiritual goals despite the physical distance.

Ultimately, building a support network requires intentionality and effort from both the men working away and their families. By nurturing these connections, they can mitigate the long-term psychological effects of separation, maintain a strong sense of identity, and uphold their values and beliefs. As they share their experiences and support one another, they create a foundation that empowers them to face the challenges of distance with grace and resilience, reinforcing the bonds of faith and family that are integral to their lives.

Developing Independence and Self-Care

In the context of Christian men working far from home, developing independence and self-care becomes paramount for both the men and their families. The physical distance often leads to emotional isolation, making it crucial for these men to cultivate a sense of autonomy that helps them manage their responsibilities effectively. This independence is not only about managing daily tasks but also involves nurturing one's mental and spiritual health, which can be severely tested during prolonged separations from family. Men must learn to engage in self-care practices that allow them to recharge emotionally and spiritually, thereby enabling them to support their families from afar.

Self-care routines can take various forms, including regular exercise, prayer, and personal reflection. These activities serve as essential tools that help men cope with the stress and emotional fatigue that come with long-distance work. Regular physical activity can alleviate feelings of anxiety and promote a sense of well-being, while prayer serves as a connection to their faith, reinforcing a sense of purpose and belonging. Additionally, incorporating time for personal reflection allows these men to process their experiences, fostering a deeper understanding of their emotional landscape and the impact of their work on their family dynamics.

For wives and children, the absence of a father figure can lead to feelings of neglect and emotional instability. It is vital for families to adapt to this new dynamic by encouraging independence in their daily lives. Wives may take on new roles in managing household responsibilities, which can empower them but might also lead to feelings of resentment or isolation. Open communication about these changes is essential, as it fosters a sense of teamwork and shared responsibility, allowing both partners to thrive in their respective roles despite the distance.

Spiritual practices within the family can also be affected by the absence of the father. Families might find it challenging to maintain their usual routines of prayer and worship when one member is away. Therefore, it becomes important to establish new traditions that include virtual gatherings or shared devotional times, fostering a sense of unity despite physical separation. These practices not only keep the family spiritually connected but also serve as a reminder of their collective faith, reinforcing the values that underpin their relationships.

Finally, community support systems play a crucial role in helping families navigate the challenges of long-distance work. Churches and local groups can provide resources, encouragement, and fellowship, creating a network of understanding and support. By engaging with these communities, families can find solace and practical advice, promoting resilience in the face of adversity. As Christian men develop their independence and prioritize self-care, they can better support their families, ensuring that both they and their loved ones remain spiritually and emotionally connected, despite the challenges of distance.

Managing Household Responsibilities Alone

Managing household responsibilities alone can present a significant challenge for families where men work far from home. For wives and children, the sudden shift in dynamics can lead to feelings of overwhelm and isolation. The absence of a partner or father means that the responsibilities traditionally shared must now be navigated by one person. Household chores, financial management, and emotional support all fall on the remaining family members, often leading to stress and fatigue. The emotional toll can be heavy, especially when the absent spouse's role was crucial in maintaining household harmony.

As Christian families face these challenges, the impact on spiritual practices can be profound. Regular family prayers, devotions, and shared spiritual activities are often disrupted by distance. The absence of a father figure during these moments can lead to feelings of disconnection from faith, leaving wives and children to seek spiritual fulfilment independently. This shift can create a sense of spiritual isolation, as family members grapple with maintaining their faith without the support of their loved one. The struggle to uphold shared values and beliefs can be daunting, particularly during times of stress.

Marital strain frequently accompanies the pressures of long-distance work. Wives may feel the burden of managing not just household responsibilities, but also the emotional landscape of the family. Communication can become strained, and misunderstandings may arise due to the physical separation. Couples often find it difficult to discuss their feelings, leading to further disconnection. The emotional distance created by work-related travel can erode the foundation of trust and intimacy, resulting in conflicts that require careful navigation to preserve the marriage.

The influence of work-related travel on a Christian man's identity and values also plays a critical role in family dynamics. Men may struggle with feelings of guilt for being away from home, leading to a diminished sense of self-worth. The need to provide financially can overshadow the importance of being present emotionally and spiritually for their families. As they adapt to their roles as distant providers, the challenge lies in balancing their professional identity with their responsibilities as husbands and fathers. This can cause internal conflict and a re-evaluation of personal values, impacting their overall sense of purpose.

Community support systems become essential for families managing these challenges. Churches and local organizations can provide resources and

emotional support for wives and children left behind.
Engaging in community activities can offer a sense of
belonging and help mitigate feelings of isolation.
Additionally, fostering connections with other
families in similar situations can create networks of
understanding and shared experiences. By building a
support system, families can navigate the
complexities of distance, maintaining their faith and
resilience in the face of separation.

Chapter 9: Family Spiritual Practices Across Distances

Maintaining Family Prayer Routines

Maintaining family prayer routines is essential for Christian families, especially when the father is working away from home. Distance can create emotional isolation and a sense of disconnect, not only between the father and the family but also among family members themselves. Establishing a consistent prayer schedule can serve as a vital lifeline, helping to bridge the gap created by physical separation. Families can set specific times for prayer, ensuring that all members participate, whether through phone calls, video chats, or even group messaging. This practice reinforces a sense of unity and shared faith, allowing family members to feel connected to one another despite the miles that may separate them.

Incorporating prayer into daily routines can also provide a structured way for families to cope with the emotional challenges of separation. For wives and children, the absence of a husband and father can lead to feelings of loneliness and anxiety. Regular prayer can help alleviate these feelings by fostering a supportive environment where family members can express their worries and hopes to God. This shared spiritual practice encourages openness and vulnerability, allowing family members to feel heard and validated in their struggles. Over time, this can strengthen the overall emotional resilience of the family, helping them navigate the complexities of long-distance relationships.

Moreover, family prayer routines can play a significant role in the spiritual development of children. Children often look to their parents as models of faith, and when a father is absent, they may struggle to maintain their spiritual practices. By engaging children in prayer, mothers can help them cultivate a personal relationship with God, reinforcing the values and teachings that are central to their family's beliefs. Prayer can become a foundation for discussing spiritual matters, allowing children to ask questions and develop their understanding of faith. This practice not only nurtures their spiritual growth but also helps them feel a sense of belonging within the family unit.

Marital strain is another challenge that families with distant working fathers often face. Maintaining a strong connection through prayer can help couples address issues of communication and intimacy that may arise from physical separation. Couples can commit to praying together, even if it is through a phone call, fostering an environment of support and understanding. This shared spiritual practice can serve as an anchor for their relationship, reminding them of their commitment to one another and to God. It can also create opportunities for discussing their feelings and challenges, ultimately strengthening their bond.

Lastly, community support systems are crucial for families dealing with the unique challenges of long-distance work. Engaging with a church or faith-based community can provide additional resources for maintaining family prayer routines. These communities often offer programs and support groups that encourage families to connect, share their experiences, and pray together. By tapping into these resources, families can enhance their spiritual practices and combat the feelings of isolation that often accompany distance. The collective strength of faith communities can empower families to overcome the challenges of separation, fostering a deep sense of belonging and connection to God and one another.

Adapting Spiritual Practices for Distance

Adapting spiritual practices for distance requires intentionality and creativity, especially for Christian men who find themselves separated from their families due to work commitments. The physical absence often leads to emotional isolation, making it vital for men to maintain a strong spiritual connection despite the miles that separate them. Families can enhance their spiritual lives by incorporating technology into their routines. Virtual prayer meetings or online Bible studies can provide a platform for men to engage with their faith while remaining connected to their loved ones. This adaptation not only nurtures their spiritual growth but also reinforces familial bonds that might otherwise weaken during prolonged absences.

In addition to online gatherings, families can develop new rituals that accommodate distance. For instance, families might consider setting aside specific times for collective prayer or devotion, even if they are apart. This could involve sharing prayer requests through messaging apps or using video calls to read scripture together. Such practices help to cultivate a sense of unity and shared purpose, allowing both the men and their families to feel spiritually connected despite the challenges of physical separation. This intentional scheduling of spiritual time can also reduce feelings of guilt or anxiety about being away, as it emphasizes the importance of ongoing engagement with faith.

Moreover, the emotional toll of long-distance work relationships can sometimes lead to feelings of inadequacy or disconnection from one's spiritual identity. Men may grapple with questions about their role as spiritual leaders within the family while they are away. To adapt to these challenges, it is essential for men to find ways to express their faith individually, even in solitude. This may include personal devotions, journaling, or engaging in spiritual reading. By creating a personal spiritual practice that reflects their circumstances, men can reinforce their identity as faithful individuals, which will have a positive impact on their families as well.

The effects of distance on family prayer and spiritual practices can be profound. Traditional routines may be disrupted, leaving families feeling disjointed in their spiritual lives. However, adapting these practices can strengthen family ties and provide a sense of normalcy. Families may explore creative ways to integrate prayer into daily activities, such as praying at mealtimes or during family phone calls. These small adjustments can help keep the family spiritually grounded and encourage open discussions about faith, fostering an environment where children can continue to grow in their spiritual development.

Lastly, it is crucial for families to create a support network that fosters spiritual resilience. Connecting with other families experiencing similar challenges can provide mutual encouragement and shared resources. Community support systems, such as church groups or online forums, can offer essential connections that help mitigate feelings of isolation. By sharing experiences and strategies, families can collectively adapt their spiritual practices to better suit their unique circumstances, ensuring that faith remains a cornerstone of their lives, even when physical distance threatens to disrupt their unity.

The Importance of Shared Faith Experiences

Shared faith experiences serve as a vital connection for families who endure the challenges of distance due to work commitments. When Christian men work away from home, the absence can lead to emotional isolation not just for them, but also for their wives and children. Engaging in shared spiritual practices, such as prayer, worship, and study of scripture, can help bridge the emotional gap created by separation. These experiences foster a sense of unity and belonging, allowing families to maintain a spiritual connection that transcends physical distance.

The impact of absentee fatherhood on children's spiritual development cannot be underestimated. Children thrive in environments where they feel secure and connected to their parents, especially in their formative years. When fathers are physically absent, the risk of spiritual disconnection increases, potentially leading to confusion regarding their faith and values. However, families that prioritize shared faith experiences create opportunities for fathers to impart their beliefs and values, even from afar. This can be achieved through regular family devotionals, virtual church services, or collaborative prayer sessions, ensuring that children feel their father's presence in their spiritual lives.

Marital strain is another significant issue faced by couples separated by work. The emotional distance can lead to misunderstandings and feelings of neglect, impacting the couple's spiritual intimacy. Shared faith experiences can mitigate these effects by providing a common ground for communication and emotional support. Couples who engage in joint prayer or study scripture together, whether in person or virtually, can strengthen their bond and navigate the complexities of their relationship. This shared commitment to faith can remind couples of their shared values and goals, reinforcing their partnership even amid physical separation.

Coping with separation anxiety is critical for both men and their families. Faith can serve as a powerful tool in managing these feelings and maintaining emotional health. When families engage in shared faith practices, they create a supportive environment that fosters resilience. Regular communication about spiritual experiences and challenges can help husbands and wives feel more connected, while children can be reassured of their father's love and commitment through shared prayer and discussions about faith. This proactive approach to maintaining spiritual ties can alleviate some of the burdens associated with distance.

Community support systems also play a crucial role in sustaining shared faith experiences during times of separation. Church communities can provide a robust network for families of traveling Christian professionals, offering encouragement and resources that help maintain spiritual practices. Whether through small groups, online gatherings, or family-oriented church events, these communal experiences can reinforce the values and beliefs that families hold dear. Such support not only helps families cope with the challenges of distance but also fosters a sense of belonging and connection that is essential for nurturing faith amidst life's trials.

Chapter 10: Guilt and Responsibility

Common Feelings of Guilt Among Christian Men

Common feelings of guilt among Christian men who work away from home often stem from the inherent conflict between professional responsibilities and family obligations. These men frequently grapple with the pressure to provide financially, which can lead to neglecting their emotional and spiritual roles within the family. The guilt arises from the realization that while they fulfil their duties as providers, they are also missing essential moments in their children's lives and failing to participate in their spiritual growth. This internal struggle can create a sense of inadequacy, as they feel torn between their job's demands and their desire to be present for their families.

The emotional isolation experienced by many of these men compounds their feelings of guilt. Long-distance work often leads to a disconnection from their partners and children, making it challenging to maintain a strong family bond. As they navigate the complexities of their roles, they may feel that they are not only letting their families down but also failing to uphold their Christian values of love, commitment, and presence. This isolation can create a cycle of guilt, where the longer they are away, the more they feel responsible for the emotional toll it takes on their loved ones.

For many Christian men, the pressure to be the spiritual leader of their families adds another layer of guilt. When they are physically absent, they may worry that their children miss out on vital teachings and guidance that they would typically provide. This concern is particularly poignant when considering the potential impact on their children's spiritual development. Many men wrestle with the fear that their absence may lead to a weakened faith in their children, prompting feelings of guilt over their perceived failure as spiritual mentors.

Marital strain is another significant factor contributing to feelings of guilt among these men. The distance can exacerbate communication issues, leading to misunderstandings and conflicts that may have been manageable in person. Christian couples often rely on shared spiritual practices to maintain their connection, but when one partner is away, the absence of these rituals can lead to feelings of disconnection and resentment. Men may feel guilty for not being able to support their wives emotionally or spiritually during these challenging times, deepening their sense of responsibility for the marital strain that arises from separation.

Ultimately, the intersection of work, family, and faith creates a complex web of guilt for Christian men working away from home. They face the challenge of reconciling their professional aspirations with their roles as husbands and fathers. The desire to provide for their families while simultaneously being present for them can feel like an insurmountable burden. Many men find themselves in a constant battle against guilt, questioning their choices and their ability to live out their faith in a way that honours both their work commitments and their family responsibilities.

Navigating Expectations of Work and Family

Navigating the expectations of work and family can be particularly challenging for Christian men who find themselves working far from home. The tension between fulfilling professional obligations and maintaining family connections often leads to feelings of guilt and inadequacy. Christian men are frequently caught in a struggle to provide for their families while also nurturing their relationships, leading to emotional isolation. This disconnect can affect their self-perception and spiritual identity, as they grapple with the implications of their absence on their families and their own faith journeys.

For many families, the absence of a father figure can have profound implications for children's spiritual development. Children may experience a lack of guidance in their formative years, which can hinder their understanding of faith and moral values. Without regular interaction with their fathers, there is a risk that children may feel disconnected from the spiritual practices that are essential to their upbringing. This absence can manifest in various ways, including decreased participation in family prayer and worship, which are vital components of a Christian household. The emotional void created by an absentee father may prompt children to seek out other sources of validation, potentially leading them away from the faith.

Marital strain is another significant consequence of long-distance work relationships. The physical separation creates emotional distance, which can lead to misunderstandings and resentment between couples. Christian couples often face unique challenges as they attempt to maintain their commitment to each other while navigating the complexities of distance. Communication can suffer, and the lack of shared experiences may erode the intimacy necessary for a thriving marriage. Couples may find themselves questioning their roles and responsibilities, leading to feelings of frustration and disconnection.

Faith plays a crucial role in how families cope with the anxiety of separation. For many Christian families, turning to prayer and scripture offers solace and a sense of community. Engaging in spiritual practices can help mitigate feelings of isolation and reinforce the family unit despite physical distance. However, the challenge lies in maintaining these practices consistently, as the absence of a father can disrupt established routines. Support from church communities and fellow believers can be invaluable, providing encouragement and accountability as families navigate the emotional landscape of separation.

The long-term psychological effects of separation on Christian men can alter their life choices and perspectives. Men may grapple with feelings of failure or inadequacy, which can influence their career paths and personal relationships. The struggle to balance work and family commitments often leads to a re-evaluation of priorities, with many men questioning the value of their work in relation to their family's well-being. Ultimately, navigating the expectations of work and family requires a thoughtful approach, where open communication, faith, and community support become essential tools for fostering resilience and connection amid the challenges of distance.

Finding Balance in Responsibilities

Finding balance in responsibilities is a critical aspect for Christian men who work far from home, as they navigate the complexities of their roles both in the workplace and within their families. The demands of a job that requires significant travel often create a disconnection between men and their families, leading to feelings of guilt and emotional isolation. These men grapple with the need to provide financially while simultaneously yearning to be present for their loved ones. Understanding the importance of striking a balance can help mitigate some of the detrimental effects of long-distance work on family dynamics.

The emotional isolation experienced by many Christian men in long-distance work relationships can have profound implications for their mental health and overall well-being. As they spend extended periods away from their families, they may struggle with feelings of loneliness and disconnection. This emotional distance can lead to a diminished sense of self-worth and purpose, as their identities become intertwined with their professional obligations rather than their roles as fathers and husbands. Recognizing these feelings is the first step toward finding a healthier balance between work and home life.

Absentee fatherhood, a common outcome of frequent travel, presents significant challenges to children's spiritual development. When fathers are physically absent, their ability to impart values, engage in spiritual discussions, and model faith becomes severely limited. This absence can hinder children's understanding of their faith and diminish their sense of security within the family unit. Christian men must actively seek ways to maintain spiritual connections with their children despite the physical distance, whether through phone calls, video chats, or sending devotional materials.

Marital strain often accompanies the realities of long-distance work, as couples must navigate communication barriers and unmet emotional needs. The absence of shared experiences can create a rift in the marital relationship, leading to misunderstandings and feelings of neglect. In this context, it is vital for couples to establish intentional communication practices, set aside time for meaningful conversations, and engage in shared spiritual activities, even from afar. By prioritizing their relationship and making concerted efforts to connect, couples can strengthen their bond despite the challenges posed by distance.

Faith plays a crucial role in helping Christian families cope with the anxieties that arise from separation. In moments of loneliness and uncertainty, turning to prayer and scripture can provide comfort and guidance. Engaging in family prayer, even when physically apart, can foster a sense of unity and purpose. Furthermore, community support systems can offer additional resources and encouragement for families facing the unique struggles of long-distance work. By leaning on their faith and community, Christian men and their families can find strength in their responsibilities, ultimately creating a more balanced approach to their lives.

Chapter 11: Community Supports for Traveling Professionals

Building a Supportive Community

Building a supportive community is essential for Christian men who work far from home and their families. The emotional toll of distance can create feelings of isolation and disconnection, not only for the men themselves but also for their wives and children. A strong community can serve as a lifeline, providing encouragement, understanding, and practical assistance. When families come together to share their experiences, they can foster a sense of belonging that mitigates the loneliness often felt during prolonged separations.

In many cases, the emotional isolation that men experience while working away can lead to a disconnect from their families and their faith. Supportive communities can help bridge this gap by offering opportunities for fellowship and spiritual growth. This might include church groups, online forums, or local gatherings where families can connect with others facing similar challenges. Through these interactions, they can share coping strategies, prayer requests, and personal testimonies that reinforce their faith and strengthen their bonds.

The impact of absentee fatherhood on children's spiritual development is profound. Children may struggle with feelings of abandonment or confusion regarding their father's role in their lives. A supportive community can help mitigate these feelings by providing mentorship and guidance. Church programs designed for children of traveling parents can create a safe space for them to express their feelings, learn about faith, and build relationships with other adults who can serve as positive role models. This not only aids in their spiritual growth but also helps them feel connected despite the physical absence of their fathers.

Marital strain is another significant concern for couples separated by distance. Communication can falter under the pressures of work and life demands, leading to misunderstandings and resentment. A supportive community can offer resources for couples to maintain healthy relationships, such as workshops on effective communication and conflict resolution. Couples can also benefit from shared experiences and advice from others who have successfully navigated similar challenges, reinforcing the idea that they are not alone in their struggles.

The role of faith in coping with separation anxiety cannot be overstated. A supportive community grounded in shared beliefs can provide emotional and spiritual sustenance for families dealing with the challenges of distance. Regular group prayer and spiritual activities can help families maintain their connection to God and each other, despite physical separation. By nurturing these relationships within a supportive community, families can cultivate resilience, ensuring that their faith remains a central pillar in their lives even when distance threatens to pull them apart.

Leveraging Church Resources for Families

Leveraging church resources can be a vital strategy for families impacted by the challenges of having men work far from home. Churches often serve as community hubs that provide spiritual, emotional, and practical support. They offer various programs and resources that can help families navigate the difficulties associated with long-distance work relationships. By engaging with their church community, families can find solace in shared experiences and gain access to tools that foster resilience and connection during periods of separation.

One of the key resources that churches can offer is counselling and support groups specifically tailored for families experiencing absenteeism due to work. These groups provide a safe space for wives and children to express their feelings and share their struggles, promoting emotional well-being. Through group discussions and professional guidance, families can explore the emotional isolation that often accompanies distant work and develop coping strategies. This collective sharing can help alleviate feelings of loneliness and foster a sense of belonging, reminding families that they are not alone in their experiences.

In addition to emotional support, churches can facilitate structured family activities and events that encourage bonding despite physical distance. Regular family nights, retreats, or workshops can engage both the working men when they are home and their families while they are away. These events can foster communication, reinforce family ties, and create lasting memories, helping to mitigate the impact of separation. Such initiatives encourage families to prioritize their spiritual practices, ensuring that faith remains a central aspect of their lives, even when physical presence is lacking.

Churches also play a crucial role in providing resources for children facing the realities of absentee fatherhood. Sunday school programs, youth groups, and mentorship opportunities can help nurture children's spiritual development, offering them guidance and support in their father's absence. By engaging children in faith-based activities, churches can help them maintain a strong connection to their faith and community, which is essential for their emotional and spiritual growth. This involvement can also help children process their feelings about their father's absence, promoting resilience and a sense of stability.

Lastly, churches can serve as a platform for promoting awareness and understanding of the unique challenges faced by families of traveling professionals. By facilitating workshops and discussions on the emotional and spiritual impact of distance, churches can equip families with the tools they need to cope and thrive. This proactive approach encourages families to leverage their faith as a source of strength, allowing them to navigate their circumstances with grace and purpose. By fostering a supportive community, churches can help families transform the challenges of distance into an opportunity for deeper faith and connection.

The Importance of Connection with Others

The importance of connection with others cannot be overstated, especially for Christian men who find themselves working far from home. This separation often leads to emotional isolation, as men grapple with the challenges of maintaining relationships while fulfilling their professional obligations. The physical distance can create a psychological barrier, making it difficult for men to engage meaningfully with their families and communities. This isolation can lead to feelings of loneliness, disconnection, and even despair, which can ultimately affect their mental health and spiritual well-being.

For the wives and children left behind, the impact of distance can be profound. Wives often bear the emotional burden of single parenting, managing household responsibilities, and nurturing the spiritual growth of their children without the daily presence of their husbands. This can lead to a sense of imbalance in the family dynamic, as children may feel the absence of their father not just physically but also emotionally. The role of fathers in the spiritual development of their children is critical, and their absence can hinder the establishment of a solid foundation for faith and values within the family.

Marital strain is another significant consequence of prolonged separation. Couples may struggle to maintain intimacy and communication, which are essential components of a healthy marriage. The lack of shared experiences can create feelings of resentment or misunderstanding, as partners may feel disconnected from one another's lives. The challenges of managing a long-distance relationship require intentional effort and commitment, but without a strong connection, many couples may find it difficult to sustain their marriage under these circumstances.

Faith plays a crucial role in helping families cope with the anxiety and stress that accompany separation. Many Christian families turn to their faith communities for support, finding strength in shared beliefs and practices. Engaging in prayer, Bible study, and fellowship can help bridge the emotional gap created by distance. Families who prioritize their spiritual connection often report a greater sense of unity and resilience, as they draw on their faith to navigate the trials of separation and maintain a sense of hope.

Lastly, community support systems can be invaluable for families of traveling Christian professionals. These networks provide emotional and practical assistance, helping to alleviate feelings of isolation. By fostering connections with others who understand their struggles, families can find encouragement and resources that empower them to adapt to their unique circumstances. Building and maintaining relationships within their faith community not only enhances their spiritual lives but also reinforces their sense of belonging, providing a buffer against the emotional toll of distance.

Chapter 12: Long-Term Psychological Effects

Understanding the Psychological Impact of Separation

Separation due to work commitments often imposes a profound psychological burden on Christian men and their families. The emotional landscape changes dramatically when a husband or father is physically absent, leading to feelings of loneliness, anxiety, and emotional disconnection. Christian men may grapple with the tension between fulfilling professional responsibilities and nurturing their familial roles. This conflict can lead to a sense of inadequacy as they struggle to reconcile their work commitments with their desire to be present for their loved ones, ultimately affecting their mental well-being and self-perception.

The emotional isolation that often accompanies long-distance work can lead to significant challenges for men. The absence of daily interactions with their families can result in feelings of detachment and loneliness. This isolation can exacerbate existing insecurities and lead to a decline in mental health, as men may feel they are losing their connection to their families and their faith. Moreover, the lack of emotional support from their spouses can intensify these feelings, leading to a cycle of disconnection that impacts their overall emotional health and spiritual life.

Children, too, bear the brunt of their father's absence. The role of an absentee father can hinder their spiritual development, as children often rely on their fathers for guidance in faith-related matters. When fathers are frequently away, the spiritual dynamic within the family can shift, resulting in diminished opportunities for prayer, worship, and open discussions about faith. This absence can leave children feeling abandoned or uncertain about their spiritual journey, as they may struggle to understand the reasons behind their father's absence and its implications for their relationship with God.

Marital strain is another significant consequence of separation, particularly for Christian couples who may harbour expectations of emotional support and shared spiritual growth. The physical distance can lead to misunderstandings and resentment, as partners may feel neglected or unappreciated. The challenge of maintaining intimacy and open communication becomes paramount, and couples may find themselves navigating a complicated landscape of emotions. This strain can erode the foundation of trust and connection, making it essential for couples to actively seek ways to bridge the gap created by distance.

Faith can serve as a crucial coping mechanism for families dealing with separation. Many Christian families turn to their beliefs to find strength and solace during challenging times. Prayer, scripture, and community support can help mitigate feelings of guilt, responsibility, and loneliness. By fostering a sense of shared spiritual commitment, families can create a resilient framework that supports each member's emotional health. Additionally, developing adaptation strategies, such as setting regular communication schedules or engaging in family prayer, can help maintain connections and reinforce the family's spiritual foundation despite the challenges of physical separation.

Life Choices Influenced by Distance

Life choices influenced by distance can be profound and multifaceted, particularly for Christian men working far from home. As these men engage in long-distance work relationships, they often find themselves grappling with emotional isolation that can alter their perspectives on life and faith. The absence from their families creates a void that may lead to feelings of disconnect, prompting them to reevaluate their priorities and beliefs. This shift can manifest in various ways, including diminished engagement in church activities and a struggle to maintain spiritual practices that were once integral to their lives.

For many Christian men, the physical distance from their families and communities can contribute to a sense of guilt and responsibility that weighs heavily on their hearts. The demands of their careers often conflict with their desire to be present fathers and husbands, leading to a re-evaluation of their roles. This can impact their identity, as they may feel torn between professional obligations and family commitments. The internal struggle to balance work and family can lead to decisions that prioritize job security over spiritual fulfilment, ultimately affecting their sense of purpose and connection to their faith.

The effects of absentee fatherhood extend beyond the individual man, significantly impacting the spiritual development of children. When fathers are physically absent, children may miss out on crucial moments of guidance and support that shape their understanding of faith and moral values. This absence can lead to a disconnect from familial spiritual practices, resulting in children feeling lost or unsupported in their faith journeys. The challenge becomes not only maintaining a connection with their children but also fostering an environment where spiritual growth can thrive, despite the physical distance.

Marital strain is another critical aspect of life choices influenced by distance. The emotional toll of separation can create tension and misunderstandings between spouses, as the challenges of managing a household alone can lead to feelings of resentment and isolation. Couples may find it difficult to communicate effectively, resulting in a breakdown of intimacy and trust. This strain can lead to decisions that either strengthen the relationship through intentional efforts to reconnect or, conversely, drift apart, as the distance becomes a barrier to emotional closeness.

In navigating these complexities, faith plays a crucial role in coping with separation anxiety. Many families find solace in prayer and community support, which can help bridge the gap created by physical distance. Developing adaptation strategies is essential for wives of Christian men working away, as they often assume the role of both caregiver and spiritual leader in the absence of their husbands. Cultivating a strong support network and prioritizing family spiritual practices can help mitigate the adverse effects of distance, allowing families to maintain their faith and connection despite the challenges posed by separation.

Strategies for Healing and Growth Post-Separation

Healing and growth after a separation due to work-related distance can be a challenging journey for Christian families. One of the most effective strategies for healing is fostering open communication. Both partners should make a concerted effort to share their feelings, experiences, and daily challenges. This exchange not only builds emotional intimacy but also allows each partner to understand the other's struggles more deeply. Regular check-ins through phone calls, video chats, or even written letters can create a sense of connection, making each partner feel valued and heard despite the physical distance.

Another significant strategy is to prioritize family rituals that can be maintained across distances. This might include regular family prayer times, virtual game nights, or shared Bible study sessions. Engaging in these practices can help reinforce family bonds and maintain spiritual unity, which is crucial for Christian families. When parents are proactive in including their children in these rituals, it also sends a message of stability and love, fostering a sense of belonging and security despite the separation.

Additionally, both partners should explore personal growth opportunities during this time apart. For men working away, this could involve engaging in personal development activities such as online courses, reading, or participating in community service. For wives and children, finding local support groups or church activities can provide emotional support and social connections. Encouraging each other to grow individually can lead to a more enriched family dynamic when reunited, as each person brings new insights and experiences to the relationship.

Addressing the emotional isolation that often accompanies long-distance work is also essential. Men can benefit from connecting with other Christian men who understand their struggles, whether through online forums, church groups, or local meetups. This sense of camaraderie can help alleviate feelings of loneliness and guilt. Similarly, wives should seek community support, whether through friends, family, or church networks, to create a robust support system that helps them navigate their feelings of isolation and anxiety.

Finally, reflecting on the shared values and vision for the family can guide both partners through this transitional phase. Setting goals that align with their faith can provide direction and purpose, whether it's planning for future family activities or discussing long-term aspirations.

By grounding their journey in shared beliefs and aspirations, families can create a sense of hope and resilience, transforming the challenges of separation into opportunities for deeper connection and spiritual growth.

More About the Author

Hannes van Zyl was born in Ermelo in the mid-sixties as the first of four siblings. He grew up on farms and enjoyed a healthy childhood. During his schooling years, he lived in a hostel, returning home on weekends and holidays. With his parents often away on business, he spent weekends with his grandparents and holidays with his parents.

After completing school, he joined the Prison Service, where he worked with death row inmates at Pretoria Maximum Prison, studied Psychology, and witnessed executions. After two years, he resigned and served in Panster, Bloemfontein, participating in final operations in Angola.

In the late eighties, he worked as a salesperson in Pretoria and, in the early nineties, started a business with a friend. He relocated to Rustenburg in the mid-nineties to launch a food industry business with his parents, later becoming an estate agent and

*furthering his studies in Project Management
in the late nineties.*

*Hannes has built a solid professional
background, leading high-performing teams
with expertise in budgeting, timeline
coordination, and risk management. His
strengths include effective communication
and the ability to collaborate with cross-
functional teams while managing multiple
projects on time and within budget. With
extensive experience in construction
management, he excels in project planning
and innovative problem-solving, consistently
meeting deadlines, staying within budget, and
exceeding quality standards.*

*He is adept at stakeholder collaboration,
defining objectives, and ensuring customer
satisfaction, demonstrating a results-oriented
approach in dynamic environments.*

*In his thirties, he took on the role of a father
figure to two young men, ages 19 and 20,
which transformed his life and provided him*

with renewed purpose. He is also a proud grandfather to three grandchildren. Tragically, his eldest son passed away in a motorcycle accident in late 2023.

As a Property Practitioner, he assists sellers and buyers in marketing and purchasing properties at fair prices, prepares essential paperwork such as contracts and leases, and collaborates with attorneys and lenders to estimate property values.

As a Life Coach and Public Speaker with 20 years of experience, he has helped over 300 clients set and achieve their goals, achieving positive outcomes in 139 out of 140 suicide cases, managing 126 child abuse cases, and realizing an 80% success rate in 189 drug abuse cases. He has authored seven self-help courses and delivered numerous seminars on transformative topics.

As a Project Manager and Director, he co-planned designs for various projects, successfully completing eight estates with 595 units, all on time and within budget. He also managed the construction of ten luxury homes, overseeing landscaping for these projects.

In his roles as a Business Administrator and Project Manager, he led teams in planning significant projects like a Retirement Village costing R 195 million and a 90-bed private hospital costing R 576 million. He redesigned a plot into a wedding venue in Pretoria for R 6,500,000.

His diplomas include Project Management, Business Administration, and Structural Engineering, alongside certificates in various fields such as Engineering Management and Public Speaking.

Throughout his life, he has maintained a passion for writing. In late 2024, he decided to pursue writing full-time, aiming to complete over 15 titles he has developed, with many more ideas and stories yet to come.

More Books by the Author

Heartfelt Obedience: Discovering the Blessings of Honouring Parents

The Bible places significant emphasis on the concept of honour, particularly in the context of familial relationships. One of the most well-known commandments regarding honour is found in Exodus 20:12, which states, "Honor your father and your mother, so that you may live long in the land the Lord your God is giving you." This commandment highlights the importance of respecting and valuing one's parents. It establishes a foundational principle that underscores the relationship between children and their parents, suggesting that honouring them is not just a moral obligation but also linked to the well-being and longevity of one's life.

In addition to the commandment in Exodus, the Bible offers various verses that further elaborate on the significance of honouring parents. Proverbs 1:8 encourages children to heed the instruction of their parents, emphasizing the wisdom that can be gained from listening to them. This highlights the idea that honour goes beyond mere obedience; it encompasses actively seeking to learn from parental guidance. By embracing this principle, children can cultivate a deeper appreciation for their parents'

Enduring The Silence: Stories of Hope by Scripture

As we embark on our own journeys of patience and
trust, let us draw strength and encouragement from
these timeless stories that continue to inspire
countless individuals across generations. Each story
serves as a reminder that even in our darkest
moments, we are not alone; God walks alongside us,
guiding us through life's valleys and difficulties. Even
in those quiet moments when we might feel isolated
and uncertain, God is working in surprising and
profound ways, weaving together every experience,
challenge, and triumph into a meaningful whole.

 By choosing to move forward in faith, we align
ourselves with His divine plan, transforming our
waiting into a testament of hope and resilience that
can uplift and encourage others on their own
journeys.

Let us remember that our faith journey isn't solely for
our own benefit; it serves as a beacon of hope for
those who may be struggling to find their way in life. It
illuminates the path through darkness and inspires

others to seek truth and light in their own lives, fostering a deeper connection with the divine.

Beyond the Veil: Finding Hope after the Death of a Child

The death of a child is often regarded as the greatest tragedy one can ever experience. There is truly nothing more heartbreaking in life. In addition to the typical symptoms and stages of grief that many individuals face, various factors contribute to the unique and profound challenges of parental bereavement. The immense sorrow stemming from the loss of a child can be further complicated by a deep sense of injustice — the natural feeling that this devastating loss should never have occurred and that no parent should have to endure such pain.

Grief is an incredibly profound experience, one that touches the very core of our being in ways we often cannot articulate, especially when it involves the heartbreaking loss of a child. For many Christians, this journey through grief becomes deeply intertwined with their faith, offering a unique and transformative lens through which to understand the complexities of pain and loss. The nature of grief is multifaceted; it can elicit feelings of deep sorrow, confusion, frustration, and even anger. Yet, within these swirling emotions lies the potential for profound healing, personal growth, and a renewed sense of hope that can emerge over time. By acknowledging the intricate complexity of grief, we can begin to navigate our feelings with greater awareness while holding on to the promises and comfort found in scripture, which can guide us through even the darkest moments.

Behind Closed Doors: The Psychological Impact of Hidden Love

Understanding clandestine relationships requires delving deeply into the intricate and often tumultuous emotional landscape that accompanies loving someone who is already entangled with another person. For individuals who find themselves in such complicated situations, the initial thrill and excitement can rapidly be overshadowed by a multitude of challenges and emotional upheavals. The secrecy that is inherently woven into these relationships frequently fosters a profound sense of isolation, as lovers are compelled to navigate their intense feelings away from the prying eyes of public scrutiny. This hidden existence not only complicates the dynamics of the relationship but can also lead to a significant disconnect from one's true self, ultimately stunting personal growth and severely hindering the ability to form genuine connections with others outside the clandestine affair. The emotional toll can be substantial, leaving individuals grappling with feelings of guilt, longing, and uncertainty about their future.

Second Chances: A Journey Through Faith and Forgiveness

Understanding human fallibility is essential for everyone, regardless of age or background, as we handle the complexities of life and the myriad challenges that come with it. We are all inherently imperfect, prone to mistakes and missteps that shape our experiences. Children might stumble over their words while trying to express themselves, teenagers could make impulsive decisions that lead to valuable lessons, and adults may carry the weight of regrets from the past that inform their present choices. Yet, it is through these very imperfections that we come to appreciate the richness of our journey and the depth of our connections with one another. The Bible teaches us that all have sinned and fall short of the glory of God (Romans 3:23), highlighting our shared nature of fallibility and our collective need for understanding and forgiveness. Recognizing this profound truth allows us to embrace our human condition with grace, humility, and compassion for ourselves and others.

As we take the time to reflect on our shortcomings and the areas where we may have faltered, we also come to recognize the incredible and precious gift of grace that is bestowed upon us. God's grace is defined as unmerited favour, a divine love that forgives and restores us, even in the face of our many flaws and imperfections. In our daily lives, this grace manifests itself through the forgiveness we extend not only to ourselves but also to others around us. When we choose to truly embrace forgiveness, we create a vital space for healing and personal growth. Ephesians 4:32 serves as a powerful reminder for us to be kind and compassionate, urging us to forgive one another just as in Christ, God forgave us. This profound call to forgive empowers us to move forward in our lives, transforming our past failures and mistakes into valuable lessons that deepen our faith and enrich our relationships with others. By accepting grace and practicing forgiveness, we embark on a journey of renewal and connection.

The Silent Struggle: Understanding and Supporting Those Considering the End

Suicidal thoughts frequently arise from a complex interplay of emotional, psychological, and situational factors that can be difficult to untangle. For individuals grappling with these thoughts, it may feel as though they are engulfed in a deep, overwhelming darkness that obscures any sense of hope or joy from their lives. Many may become convinced that they are caught in an unending cycle of pain, with no possible escape, which can intensify feelings of hopelessness and despair. It is vital to understand that these thoughts often serve as a symptom of deeper underlying issues, such as depression, anxiety, or trauma. Recognizing this connection is crucial for seeking help. Moreover, it is essential to acknowledge that these feelings can severely distort one's perception of reality, making it incredibly challenging to see any viable alternatives to the pain they are enduring, leading to a sense of isolation and helplessness that can be overwhelming.

For friends and family members of those who are grappling with suicidal thoughts, it is absolutely vital to approach the situation with deep empathy and compassion. Many individuals may not openly share their feelings, which can lead loved ones to feel helpless and uncertain in how to provide the necessary support. It is essential to cultivate an environment where open and honest conversations about mental health can take place without fear of judgment or stigma. By encouraging individuals to freely express their thoughts and feelings, we can *help demystify their experiences and create a safe space for vulnerability that may provide an invaluable opportunity for genuine connection. This connection can serve as a lifeline, reminding those who are in distress that they are not alone in their struggles and that there are people who care deeply about them.*

In His Image: Discovering Personal Worth through Faith

Identity is an intricate and multi-faceted concept, shaped by a wide array of elements including personal experiences, core beliefs, and evolving perspectives over time. When considering the aspect of faith, identity transcends the mere social labels we might adopt; it is profoundly influenced by our intimate connection with God. For those of us grappling with profound questions surrounding our worth and purpose in life, recognizing ourselves as being made in God's image provides a foundational and transformative perspective. This divine image not only bestows upon us a sense of intrinsic value and dignity but also inspires us to embrace our unique identities in a manner that is both deeper and more meaningful. It encourages each of us to embark on a fulfilling journey of self-discovery and personal exploration through the enriching lens of spirituality, which, in turn, deepens our connections with God and with one another in a significant way. This journey invites us to reflect on our beliefs and experiences, fostering a richer understanding of ourselves and our place in the world.

Understanding spiritual identity requires a profound and nuanced exploration of the intricate relationship between personal beliefs and the teachings of various faiths. When individuals pose the question, "Who am I in the eyes of God?" they embark on a transformative journey of self-discovery that transcends societal measures of success, achievement, and value. This significant exploration is often profoundly informed by scriptural teachings, which emphasize the vital importance of recognizing oneself as a cherished creation of God. Embracing this perspective nurtures a stronger connection to one's spiritual identity and enables us to fully embrace our authentic selves. As we navigate the complexities of life, this understanding empowers us to live with greater clarity, purpose, and fulfilment, leading to a richer engagement with both our inner selves and the broader world around us. Through this journey, individuals can cultivate a deeper appreciation for their unique spiritual paths and foster meaningful connections with others, enhancing their overall sense of belonging and purpose in the divine tapestry of existence.

Surrendering to God: Embracing Peace Through Serious Health Challenges

The moment a life-threatening diagnosis is delivered can feel like a rupture in reality, shattering the world as you know it into countless fragments. For parents, friends, and loved ones, the initial shock can quickly spiral into a whirlwind of emotions—fear, disbelief, anger, and profound sorrow. It is entirely natural to feel overwhelmed, grappling with questions that seem utterly unanswerable. In this heart-wrenching moment of crisis, it is essential to remember that you are not alone in this journey. The Lord walks with you in your darkest hours, offering strength, guidance, and comfort through His word. Leaning into your faith during this tumultuous time can be a source of profound peace, reminding you that even amidst the chaos and uncertainty, God reigns supreme and is ever-present in your life. Trust that He is there to carry you through the storm.

As you navigate the tumultuous waters of a serious illness, it may be immensely beneficial to turn to Scripture for both guidance and solace during this challenging time. Verses that speak to God's unwavering presence, such as Psalm 46:1—"God is our refuge and strength, an ever-present help in trouble"—can provide the profound reassurance needed to face the myriad challenges that lie ahead. Embracing these powerful words can truly transform your perspective, allowing you to see your circumstances not merely as a trial to endure, but as a unique opportunity for deeper reliance on God's promises and faithfulness. Engaging in Biblical meditation can further enhance this vital process, helping to quiet the storm within and anchor your spirit in His lasting peace, providing you with strength and comfort during difficult days.

The Dynamic Property Landscape: Strategies for Success in a Changing Market

The South African property market presents a complex landscape shaped by a myriad of factors that affect both residential and commercial real estate. This market is defined by its dynamic nature, with constant shifts in regulations, economic conditions, and property trends. Real estate agents, landlords, and buyers must remain acutely aware of these changes to navigate successfully. The evolving legal framework, often influenced by local government policies, plays a critical role in shaping market conditions, impacting everything from property valuations to investment strategies.

In recent years, fluctuations in the economy have contributed to a volatile property market. The repo rate, set by the South African Reserve Bank, serves as a crucial indicator of borrowing costs, directly influencing mortgage rates and, consequently, buyer affordability. As interest rates rise or fall, the demand for properties can shift dramatically. Buyers must stay informed about these changes, as understanding the implications of repo rate adjustments can significantly affect their purchasing decisions and overall market engagement.

Distance and Disconnection: The Hidden Struggles of Christian Men Away from Home

The modern work landscape has undergone significant changes, particularly with the rise of globalization and technological advancement. Many Christian men find themselves in roles that require them to travel extensively or relocate for work, often resulting in physical separation from their families. This shift has created a unique set of challenges, as these men grapple with the demands of their careers while attempting to maintain their roles as husbands and fathers. The distance can lead to emotional isolation, making it difficult for them to stay engaged with their families and uphold their spiritual commitments, which are central to their identities.

For families of Christian men working far from home, the impact of absentee fatherhood is profound. Children may struggle with feelings of abandonment, while wives often bear the burden of managing household responsibilities alone. This dynamic can hinder children's spiritual development, as they miss out on the guidance and presence of their fathers during formative years. The absence of a father figure can lead to confusion regarding faith and values, ultimately affecting the family's overall spiritual health. The challenge lies in maintaining a sense of unity and shared faith, even when physical presence is compromised

The Power Dynamics: Exploring the Top and Bottom Division

The concept of "top" and "bottom" within the gay community often extends far beyond the simplistic notion of mere sexual roles, encompassing a much broader spectrum of identity, power dynamics, and interpersonal relationships. For many individuals within the gay community, these labels can carry a significant amount of weight, profoundly influencing not only how they perceive themselves but also how they are perceived by others in social contexts. The binary classification of these roles can create an environment laden with expectations and pressures, where individuals may feel an obligation to conform to specific roles based on various factors, including their personality traits, physical appearance, or age. This societal perspective can lead to a limited and narrow understanding of identity, ultimately constraining personal expression and authenticity, thereby inhibiting individuals from fully exploring and embracing their true selves.

Growing up, many gay individuals face an overwhelming barrage of perceptions from both within and outside the gay community. Young gay individuals often feel intense pressure to conform to societal archetypes of being a "top" or a "bottom," which are frequently dictated by stereotypes that associate certain personality traits and behaviours with these roles. For instance, those who are perceived as more feminine may be pushed toward the bottom role, while those who exhibit more masculine traits are often expected to take on the top role. This societal pressure can create a profound sense of dissonance for those who do not naturally align with these stereotypes, leading to internalized homophobia, feelings of inadequacy, and a struggle with self-identity. The societal call to "be yourself" can feel profoundly contradictory when societal norms impose such rigid and limiting expectations. This dissonance can further complicate the journey of self-acceptance for many young gay individuals.

When Shadows Wisper: Embracing the Devil's Bargain

Understanding the Devil's Bargain often requires a deep dive into the motivations that drive individuals to make choices that seem counterintuitive. It's essential to recognize that this concept is not solely about succumbing to temptation but also about the complex interplay of circumstances, desires, and the human spirit's resilience. Each of us faces moments when the allure of an easier path beckons, especially when we feel abandoned or isolated. Acknowledging this temptation is the first step toward empowerment, allowing us to choose wisely rather than out of desperation.

In many narratives, the Devil's Bargain symbolizes a moment of weakness, a choice made in the heat of turmoil. However, it is crucial to reframe this understanding. Life can often feel like a series of trials, and in those moments, we may feel that all hope is lost. The devil, represent the struggles we face—fear, loneliness, and despair. Yet, it is within this darkness that we can find the strength to rise *above the challenges. Embracing the struggle can lead to profound personal growth and a deeper understanding of our values and what we truly hold dear.*

www.ingramcontent.com/pod-product-compliance
Lightning Source LLC
Chambersburg PA
CBHW051748250726
48659CB00001B/302